Simplifying Nutritional Wealth Series

A series of small, easy to read books addressing common health issues women tend to have through their years.
I have decided to mainly deal with WOMEN because we seem to throw hormones into the mix of everyday life. A lot of what we deal with and how we deal with obstacles comes from an emotional view. All we need to do is grab a hold of our hormones, keep them in balance and POOF…problem solved.

If we can understand the dynamics of controlling these hormones with nutrition, women will completely control the world they live in!! ENJOY!! Isra Girgrah Wynn

ISBN: 978-1-312-04759-4

http://www.iwynn.net

Acknowledgements:
Thank you to everyone who supports
my vision, especially my loving
husband, Marty Wynn. And thanks to
my children who keep me on my toes
24/7.

The ROOT of Healthy Hair

There are many causes of hair issues that might not be helped/treated. Some include genetics, pregnancy, aging, and stress. Others, which may be helped/treated, include hormones, anemia, prescription drugs, thyroid problems, lack of sleep and nutrient deficiencies.

The appearance of our skin, nails, & hair is one of the best indicators of our overall health. But many of us spend a ton of time and money attempting to enhance our beauty from the outside in. Some products can help some of your beauty concerns such as frizzy hair, brittle nails, or skin blemishes, but it's not a permanent fix. Research shows that a balanced, whole foods diet, rich in antioxidants, and essential vitamins and minerals such as Zinc, Biotin, Omega 3 fatty acids and Vitamins A, C, and B can help improve the health and appearance of your skin, hair, and nails.

Healthy looking hair, skin and nails are in general a sign of good health and good hair care practices. Most healthy individuals have adequate nutrients in their diet; however some people do not have access to good nutrition, others have medical illnesses that predispose them to nutritional deficiency which influence scalp/body/hair.

Nutrition is a complex subject - the effects of correct nutrition are indirect and often slow to appear. Hair in particular is slow to respond to any stimulus. Trials have indicated that correct nutrition is instrumental in healthy hair growth, and conversely many deficiencies correlate with hair loss. Hair nutrition is therefore a vital part of any treatment regime. A truly systematic and rigorous approach must be taken when formulating a nutrition supplement for hair due to the many factors that affect the eventual efficacy of the treatment.

Malnutrition, congenital heart disease, neuromuscular disease, chronic illnesses, malignancy, alcoholism, and advanced age can cause hair to change color, be weakened, or lost.

Proper nutrition is important. The living part of hair is under the scalp skin where its root is housed within its follicle. It derives its nutrients from blood. Health concerns e.g. stress, trauma, medications, medical conditions, heavy metals, smoking etc. can affect the hair.

Hair is the fastest growing natural tissue in the human body: the average rate of growth is 1 cm per month. The speed of hair growth varies based on genetics, gender, age, and hormones. It may be reduced by nutrient deficiency (i.e., anorexia, anemia, zinc deficiency) and hormonal fluctuations (i.e., menopause, polycystic ovaries, thyroid disease).

It is important to mention that many of the metabolic requirements of follicle cells (minerals and vitamins) must be satisfied for optimal hair growth. People with certain nutritional deficiencies tend to have dry, stringy and dull hair, and sometimes experience hair loss. Fortunately the latter can be restored once the deficiency is addressed.

Thinning hair and hair loss are common in men and women. Reasons range from simple and temporary - a vitamin deficiency - to the more complex like an underlying health condition.
In many cases, there are ways to treat both male and female hair loss. It all depends on the cause.

Genetics and health are factors in hair wellbeing. Genetics might be a component of female hair loss. Usually there is a strong history of baldness in the family. But genetics might only hold part of the responsibility.
Nutrition, hormone balance and stress will also play important roles. Clinically,

many women will report their hair loss started after a time of great stress. Stress that goes on for several days to months (no longer) can induce significant changes in the immune system, how well we digest and even how well we sleep. Hair loss can occur as the immune system overreacts in the area of the hair follicle. Major stress may play a significant role in this overreaction of the immune system. Any kind of physical trauma - surgery, a car accident, or severe illness, even flu - can cause temporary hair loss. This can trigger a type of hair loss called Telogen Effluvium. Hair has a programmed life cycle: growth phase, rest phase and shedding phase. When you have a really stressful event, it can shock the hair cycle, (pushing) more hair into the shedding phase. Hair loss often becomes noticeable 3-6 months after the trauma.

Emotional stress is less likely to cause hair loss than physical stress, but it can happen, for instance, in the case of divorce, after the death of a loved one, or while caring for an aging parent. More often, though, emotional stress won't actually precipitate the hair loss. It will exacerbate a problem that's already there.

The good news is that hair will start to grow back as your body recovers from physical stress. While it's not known if reducing stress can help your hair, it can't hurt either. Take steps to combat stress and anxiety like getting exercise, trying talk therapy, or getting more support if you need it. Get involved with exercises and events that help you de-stress your body.

Stress depletes vitamins and minerals therefore contributing to deficiencies in the body.

Sleep is a must have to help fight hair loss. Lack of quality, deep sleep cuts away the time frame the body uses to repair itself. Going to bed late will affect the body's healing ability. Going to bed with lights on or with ambient light from outside will also limit one's quality of sleep. Hair loss may be one of many symptoms that occur when the body is withheld from deep sleep that it needs. Plan to rest at a consistent time in a comfortable bed. When going to sleep, allow the room to be as dark as possible using blackout shades on the windows (or on eyes) as necessary.

Certain classes of **medications** may also promote hair loss. More common among them are certain blood thinners and the blood-pressure drugs known as beta-blockers. Other drugs that might cause hair loss include methotrexate (used to treat rheumatic conditions and some skin conditions), lithium (for bipolar disorder), non-steroidal anti-inflammatory drugs (NSAIDs) including ibuprofen, and possibly antidepressants. It's important to review any medications you take and discuss their potential side effects with your general practitioner and pharmacist. When hair loss does occur from a medication you're taking, there is a good chance that the hair will grow back on its own after you stop taking it. You can also talk with your doctor about the hair loss and consulting about changing the dose or switching to another medicine.

There is no solution to **aging** effects. Even with outstanding nutrition, genetic blueprint is eventually going to take control and hair may change color, structure, and density. Control of biological aging may be influenced by antioxidants and **super-foods** e.g. super-green mixes, chlorella, spirulina, micro-algae extracts such as Astaxanthin, broccoli sprouts, fresh vegetables, blueberries, raspberries, strawberries, blackberries, etc. also garlic, ginger, and other culinary and medicinal herbs. Water is important in general bodily health and potentially good hair health. **Water** quenches thirst and aids food digestion.

A hormone imbalance is just as likely to feed fear and erode self-confidence, as it is to contribute to hair loss.

Hormones can play a significant role in the health and quality of the hair. Low levels of **thyroid hormone** can be very common reason for hair loss. The thyroid gland should be evaluated closely for any signs of deficiency by both lab tests and symptom evaluation. The thyroid gland needs minerals such as iodine, zinc, and selenium to work effectively. If stress has been an issue, cortisol levels should also be evaluated. Cortisol is a hormone made in both men and women by the adrenal gland. This gland was made to respond rapidly to stress, but only in spurts, not in long sequences like those we face today. Chronic stress will eventually weaken this gland and the body. Cortisol levels can provide assessments on how well the adrenal gland is currently able to keep up. Chronic stress must be addressed and the adrenal gland must be fed to maintain the health of the body, including the health of the hair and scalp.

For both the health of the hair and for stress, Vitamin C and B complex can be very important. Throwing out the soft drinks, processed foods, sugar and artificial sweeteners will greatly improve the chances of hair follicle stimulation.

Hypothyroidism is the medical term for having an under active thyroid gland which accounts for the majority of thyroid disease cases. This little gland located in your neck produces hormones that are critical to metabolism as well as growth and development and, when it's not pumping out enough hormones, can contribute to hair loss and brittle nails among other symptoms. Synthetic thyroid medication will take care of the problem however; nutrition can also correct the issue. Once your thyroid levels return to normal, so should your hair.

Be careful; if left untreated, hypothyroidism can lead to obesity, joint pain, infertility, goiter, and heart disease because the symptoms can mimic other diseases where people do not realize that it is thyroid disease. Hypothyroidism is most often caused by an iodine-deficient diet.

Hyperthyroidism is an overactive thyroid in which your body produces too much thyroid hormone. This could lead to many symptoms including fine, brittle hair.

Hormones affect the absorption of nutrients, the body's growth processes, and nearly all aspects of health, so it is important to pursue and maintain optimum hormone balance to keep your hair healthy.

As with virtually every bodily function, your diet plays a role in the health of your thyroid. There are some specific nutrients that your thyroid depends on and it's important to include them in your diet.

Iodine: Without sufficient iodine, your thyroid cannot produce adequate hormones to help your body function on an optimal level. Because iodized salt is heavily processed, avoid salt and instead get iodine naturally from sea vegetables such as seaweed (hijiki, wakame, arame, dulse, nori, and kombu).

Selenium: Critical for the proper functioning of your thyroid gland. Can be found in foods such as shrimp, snapper, tuna, cod, halibut, calf's liver, button and shiitake mushrooms and Brazil nuts.

Zinc, Iron and Copper: These metals are needed in trace amounts for your healthy thyroid function. Foods such as calf's liver, spinach, mushrooms, turnip greens, and Swiss chard can help provide these trace metals in your diet.

Omega-3 fats: These essential fats , which are found in fish or fish oil, play an important role in thyroid function.

Coconut oil: Coconut oil is made up of mostly medium chain fatty acids, which may help to increase metabolism and promote weight loss, along with providing other thyroid benefits. This is especially beneficial for those with Hypothyroidism.

Antioxidants and B vitamins: The antioxidant vitamins A, C and E can help your body neutralize oxidative stress that may damage the thyroid. In addition, B vitamins help manufacture thyroid hormone and play an important role in healthy thyroid function.

There are certain foods that should be avoided to protect your thyroid. **Aspartame** - sweetener (NutraSweet), **Gluten** (found in wheat, rye, barley, along with most processed food). Too much **non-fermented SOY, including some soymilk, tofu, soy nuts and soy protein isolates,** may interfere with the function of the thyroid gland.

Everyone is in the process of growing and losing hair. Even the fullest head of hair loses anywhere from 50-150 hairs a day. Your **hormones** play a very large role in the process of hair growth. Many women commonly notice that their hair is at its fullest during times of **pregnancy**. After the pregnancy period, many lose large amounts of hair in short periods of time. This is a process called telogen effluvium and is a great example of the role of hormones in hair loss.

Hair loss in women is most often associated with an imbalance of estrogen and testosterone in their bodies. This often happens during times of menopause.

Factors that increase the likelihood of hair loss in women are the following:

- Use of birth control pills throughout life.
- High stress and poor posture and breathing patterns.
- Poor diet that is loaded with toxins and is deficient in essential nutrients.
- Lack of regular exercise.

- Heavy exposure to environmental toxins.

Making dietary changes is the very best first step for someone to stop this process and naturally to balance hormones. Begin adding phytonutrient dense **super foods** that are loaded with anti-oxidants, trace minerals, healthy fats and protein sources.

Three critical nutrients for healthy skin include silica, zinc, and biotin. These minerals are found in many plant and animal foods. **Silica** helps the body absorb vitamins and minerals more effectively. It is critical for healthy hair as we age and can be found in cucumbers, celery, sprouts, and bell peppers.
One of the most common nutrient deficiencies in our society today is zinc.

Zinc plays a critical role in the formation of important hormones and enzymes. Dietary phytic acids bind to zinc and reduce their effectiveness in the body. Heavy intake of dietary phylates present in many grains, legumes, and nuts is a common cause for zinc deficiencies. A lack of zinc causes the increase in a chemical messenger called Tumor Necrosis Factor alpha (TNF-a). TNF-a causes the immune system to attack healthy tissues in the body such as hair. Sufficient levels of zinc help preserve healthy hair; however, heavy doses of zinc supplementation can reverse the process and cause accelerated hair loss.

Biotin (vitamin B7) is commonly referred to as vitamin H because of its importance in producing healthy hair. Excessive consumption of alcohol, refined foods and egg whites, as well as long-term antibiotic usage can deplete the body's biotin levels.

Poor protein digestion can also be a major factor in hair loss. High stress and poor diet over time can cause a reduction in the stomach's ability to secrete hydrochloric acid. When this happens the stomach cannot lower its pH effectively enough to completely metabolize protein. Using apple cider vinegar and/or digestive enzymes in conjunction with protein foods can dramatically help.

Here are some suggestions to help keep blood sugar and hormones in balance.

- Eat regular meals without skipping meals.
- Cut down on refined and high glycemic index carbohydrates.
- Consume whole grains in moderation.
- Eat a wide variety of fresh fruits and vegetables daily.
- Eat healthy fats each day.
- Protect your body with antioxidants (they combat

cellular damage from free radicals).

Crash diets cause temporary hair loss due to incumbent nutritional factors e.g. anorexia, bulimia, and other medical conditions. Diets should contain protein, fruits, vegetables, grains, and an appropriate amount of fat. Deficiency will typically show in the hair. A mild case of anemia can cause shedding of hair. B group vitamins are significantly important for healthy hair, especially biotin. While not all hair growth issues originate from malnutrition, it is a valuable symptom in diagnosis. Crash diets with rapid weight loss can affect the normal hair cycle causing increased shedding within 6-12 weeks. This temporary problem should recover with dietary improvements.

Almost one in 10 women aged 20 - 49 suffers from **anemia** due to an iron deficiency (the most common type of anemia), which is an easily fixable cause of hair loss. Your doctor will have to do a blood test to determine for sure if you have this type of anemia.

Vitamins and minerals are the nutrients that are found in foods we eat. Your body needs them to grow, develop and work properly. When it comes to vitamins, each one has a special role to play. For example, folic acid is necessary for DNA synthesis and very important in the making of red and white blood cell production. Vitamin B12 is also needed for blood cell production as well as for maintaining healthy nerves. B vitamins in general help your body make protein and energy. In addition to vitamin B12 and folic acid, you also need iron on order to produce healthy red blood cells. Red blood cells carry oxygen from your lungs to all the parts of your body.

An often, overlooked factor is the **circulation** of oxygen and nutrients to the hair. Even a perfectly balanced supplement would be ineffective without adequate blood flow to the hair. Therefore it may be beneficial to increase circulation.

Foods that help increase blood circulation include oranges (Vitamin C), Dark chocolate (Cocoa - flavonoids), cayenne pepper (increase metabolism), Garlic (cleanses blood), ginkgo biloba (dilates blood vessels - increases blood flow), watermelon (lycopene), salmon and avocados (omega-3), sunflower seeds (vitamin E), and goji berries (fiber).

The best way to get your vitamins, minerals, proteins and fats for healthy hair is to eat a variety of the foods rich in these nutrients. The second way is to supplement daily. Here are those nutrients and the foods that contain them as well as suggestions to daily supplemental dosages. Remember to consult with your doctor when starting a new nutrition or fitness program. Everyone is different and unique in his or her own way so one program might only fit one person. Everyone has different and specific needs for their optimal health.

Healthy hair requires good nutrition, involving a wide variety of vitamins, trace minerals, amino acids, and essential fatty acids. As a result, poor nutrition will have a fairly immediate and obvious effect on hair health. Starvation dieting, rapid weight loss, and eating disorders often trigger some hair breakage or hair loss. Sometimes just introducing different foods into your diet, such as eating a lot of fried foods over a period of days when you're not used to it, can change the appearance and health of your hair.

Improper digestion is another factor that can contribute to hair loss. A lack in Pepsin (as enzyme essential for protein digestion) will interfere with the absorption of key nutrients. To have healthy hair, all eight essential amino acids are required. The hair, being mostly protein, will readily reflect poor protein status. Many elderly people have problems with digestion, which can accelerate age-related hair loss.

The essential omega-3 fatty acids, protein, vitamin B12, and iron, found in fish sources, prevent a dry scalp and dull hair color.

Dark green vegetables contain high amounts of vitamins A and C, which help with production of sebum and provide a natural hair conditioner.

Legumes provide protein to promote hair growth and also contain iron, zinc and biotin.

Biotin functions to activate certain enzymes that aid in metabolism of carbon dioxide as well as protein, fats, and carbohydrates. A deficiency in biotin intake can cause brittle hair and can lead to hair loss. In order to avoid a deficiency, individuals can find sources of biotin in cereal-grain products, liver, egg yolk, soy flour, and yeast.

Nuts contain high sources of selenium and therefore are important for a healthy scalp.

Alpha-linoleic acid and zinc are also found in some nuts and help condition the hair and prevent hair shedding that can be caused by a lack of zinc. Protein deficiencies or low-quality protein can produce weak and brittle hair, and can eventually result in loss of hair color.

Low-fat dairy products are good sources of calcium, a key component for hair growth. A balanced diet is necessary for a healthy scalp and hair. Healthy hair growth requires a complexity of nutrients and a ready supply of oxygen but comparatively few authoritative studies have trialed ingredients to maintain or promote hair growth. However, a balanced bioavailable formula to protect and maintain hair growth is vital.

A good multivitamin can be a foundation of health and nutrition. Changes in skin and hair can provide clues to the presence of an underlying vitamin deficiency.

Hair ultimately reflects the overall condition of the body. In health problems or nutritional deficiencies hair may stop growing or become brittle. If a body is in good health, it is possible to maximize genetic growth cycle through taking the proper blend of amino acids and B-vitamins.

Certain vitamins, minerals and amino acids are crucial to the metabolic pathways involved in keratin protein hair metabolism, leading to a potential loss of hair and substantial degradation of hair health.

Vitamin B5 (pantothenic acid) gives hair flexibility, strength and shine and helps prevent hair loss and greying.

Vitamin B6 helps prevent dandruff and can be found in cereals, egg yolk, and liver.

Vitamin B12 helps prevent the loss of hair and can be found in fish, eggs, chicken, and milk. It is also important to include B6, biotin, inositol and folic acid in supplemental program. It has been found that certain minerals including magnesium, sulfur, silica and zinc are also very important toward maintaining healthy hair.

Reduced levels of **thiamin** (vitamin B1), **riboflavin** (vitamin B2), **niacin**, and **pantothenic acid** can contribute to the undernourishment of hair-follicle cells. A dosage range of 25-50 mg daily is recommended.

A decrease in **folic acid** may contribute to decreased hair-follicle cell division and growth. Folic acid is also essential for the maintenance of healthy methionine levels in the body. Signs of folic-acid deficiency include anemia, apathy, fatigue, and greying hair. A therapeutic dose of 400-800 mcg daily is recommended.

Biotin, part of the vitamin B complex, is another nutrient associated with hair loss. Biotin is required for a number of enzymatic reactions within the body, and is necessary for the proper metabolism of protein, fat, and carbohydrates. Over time, poor metabolism of nutrients can contribute to undernourished hair follicle cells.

Although rare, a biotin deficiency results in skin rashes and hair loss. A study conducted at Harvard University suggests that biotin is one of the most important nutrients for preserving hair strength, texture, and function.

People who are eating adequate amount of protein should not have a problem with biotin deficiency, though vegans may be at risk. Good food sources of biotin are eggs, liver and soy. The recommended dosage of d-biotin is 500-1000 mcg per day. Other food sources include peanuts, almonds, sweet potatoes, eggs, onions, oats, tomatoes, carrots, and salmon.

One of **vitamin C**'s major functions is to help produce and maintain healthy collagen, the connective tissue type found within hair follicles. Vitamin C is also a strong antioxidant and protects both the cells found within follicles and cells in nearby blood vessels. A daily dose of 100-200 mg of vitamin C is recommended for hair and skin care. Vitamin C with bioflavonoids - one to two grams daily.

Vitamin E helps to maintain the integrity of cell membranes of hair follicles. The vitamin provides physical stability to cell membranes and acts as an antioxidant while promoting healthy skin and hair. A daily dose of vitamin E should be within the therapeutic range of 50-400 IU. Vitamin E and selenium work together to prevent attacks on cell membranes by free radicals by reducing peroxide concentration in the cell.

Beta-carotene is also important to hair growth. This is so because beta-carotene is converted to vitamin A as the body needs it, helps maintain normal growth and bone development, protective sheathing around nerve fibers, as well as promoting healthy skin, hair and nails. Dosage for beta-carotene is 10,000 to 15,000 IU daily.

Antioxidants Vitamin A, C, and E enhance skin cell turnover and collagen synthesis. When applied topically these vitamins protect against premature skin aging from the damaging effects of ultraviolet light and environmental pollutants. Foods rich in antioxidants include berries (straw, black, blue, cran, rasp), artichoke hearts, walnuts, pecans, coffee, and ground cloves.

Vitamin C helps reduce the damage caused by free radicals and UV exposure. Over time, free radicals damage collagen and elastin, the fibers that support skin structure.

Vitamin E also helps reduce the skin effects of free radicals and UV exposure. Food sources include sunflower seeds, almonds, spinach, Swiss chard, avocado, and peanuts.

Selenium is necessary for iodine metabolism. Case studies have indicated that selenium deficiency can lead to poor hair growth. Supplementation of 25-50 mcg of selenium per day is the recommended dosage.

Trace elements

Calcium - a fraction of the body's calcium stimulates cell mediators that act on cell-membrane phospholipids in hair-follicle cells. Most Americans fail to meet the recommended daily intake for calcium. Patients have to be advised to take **magnesium** with supplemental calcium to maintain healthy calcium levels in the body. Without extra magnesium to balance it, large doses of calcium may be harmful. The recommended dosage is 100-200 mg of calcium per day.

Zinc is essential for DNA and RNA production, which in turn, leads to normal follicle-cell division. zinc is also responsible for helping to stabilize cell-membrane structures and assists in the breakdown and removal of superoxide radicals. Zinc intake is generally low. Topical applications of zinc have been shown to reduce the hair loss activity of 5-AR type II. The recommended dosage is 15 mg of zinc (in the form of zinc amino acid chelate) per day. Zinc deficiencies, and any associated hair health, may associate with low-calorie diets, especially young women.

Zinc is found in meat, eggs, and seafood.

Iron deficiency causes microcytic and hypo-chromic anemia. Moreover, most other organs including the skin and pilosebaceous follicles are affected.

Iodine - Suboptimal thyroid functioning can lead to abnormal hair growth. Because iodine supports proper thyroid functioning, 112-225 mcg of iodine (in the form of kelp) per day is the recommended dosage.

Amino Acids

L-Methionine - one of four sulfur-containing amino acids, supports hair strength by providing adequate amounts of sulfur to hair cells. Sulfur is required for healthy connective tissue formation. Hair requires sulfur for normal hair growth and appearance. Food sources include eggs, fish, nuts, seeds, and green leafy veggies.

L-Cysteine - supports hair strength by the provision of sulfur. Skin, nails, and hair are high in L-Cysteine. There is evidence that deficiency may be a factor on hair loss. Supplementing the diet accordingly may be helpful. Food sources include pork, poultry, eggs, red peppers, garlic, and oats.

L-Lysine - It is interesting to note that male pattern baldness is less common in Asians than Americans. Is this in part due to the Asian diet being rich in L-Lysine - an enzyme inhibiting amino acid in vegetables and herbs affecting 5-alpha-reductase is some way.

Food sources include eggs, meat, soy, beans, and cheese.

Polyunsaturated fatty acids (PUFU's) - help reduce dry, scaly skin. Most popular sources are walnuts, fish oil, and flaxseed oil.

People on low-fat and non-fat diets are at risk for nutrition-related hair loss because hair needs essential fatty acids. Essential fatty acid deficiency causes a drying-up of the scalp and skin. These are vital nutrients that support follicular health. When the follicle is not healthy, hair loss or thinning occurs.

Tips to fighting hair loss:
- Make sure you check iron, thyroid, cortisol and vitamin D levels.
- Begin taking high potency multivitamin/multi-mineral.
- Be sure to get 1,000 - 2,000 mg of vitamin C and 5,000 mcg biotin per day.
- Take a B complex 1-2 times a day. Higher doses tend to be better for those with more stress.
- Cut out the refined sugars, sweets and processed foods.
- Eat more fruits, vegetables, and a variety of good quality proteins.
- Consider more exercise, yoga, hobbies or counseling to help the body better cope with stress.

Most hair loss can be corrected if the cause can be identified – and the sooner, the better – but proper testing is essential. Guessing based on symptoms can make matters worse or lead to a misdiagnosis because an excess of a nutrient or hormone can sometimes generate the same symptoms as a deficiency. Work with your healthcare practitioner and trichologist to determine the cause, and you are more likely to find an effective treatment.

The **Reference Daily Intake** or **Recommended Daily Intake** (**RDI**) is the daily intake level of a nutrient that is considered to be sufficient to meet the requirements of 97–98% of healthy individuals in every demographic in the United States (where it was developed, but has since been used in other places).

The RDI is used to determine the **Daily Value** (**DV**) of foods, which is printed on nutrition facts labels in the United States and Canada, which is regulated by the Food and Drug Administration (FDA).

Consult with your physician or doctor before starting or stopping a nutritional or fitness program or medications.

APPENDIX A

Healthy Hair Foods

Salmon and Mackerel provide omega-3 fatty acids, protein, Vitamin B12 and iron. Essential omega-3 fatty acids support scalp health. Deficiency can result in a dry scalp and dull hair. Vegetarians may source plant-based omega-3 fats from ground flaxseed, macadamia nuts and walnuts.

Spinach, broccoli and Swiss chard, provide vitamins A and C used in sebum production (secreted by hair follicles). Other foods rich in vitamin C include bell peppers, chili peppers, kale, guava, kiwi, berries, papaya, citrus fruits, peas, and tomatoes.

Dark green vegetables provide iron and calcium.

Beans: Legumes (kidney beans and lentils) provide protein, iron, zinc, and biotin. Biotin deficiencies can result in brittle hair.

Nuts: Brazil nuts are a natural source of selenium. Walnuts contain zinc and alpha-linoleic acid, an omega-3 fatty acid that may help hair condition. Pecans, cashews and almonds also contain zinc. Zinc deficiency can lead to hair shedding.

Poultry provides the high-quality protein and iron with a high degree of bioavailability. Weak brittle hair may derive from protein deficiency.

Eggs are sources of protein, biotin, and vitamin B12 – important beauty nutrients.

Fortified whole grain breakfast cereals, containing zinc, iron, and B vitamins are important.

Oysters provide zinc – a powerful antioxidant. In addition to other sources e.g. whole grains, nuts, beef, and lamb.

Low-fat Dairy products: calcium, whey, and casein are important minerals for hair growth sourced from skimmed milk and yogurt.

Carrots are an excellent source of vitamin A – antioxidants that work to condition and moisturize the sebum in the scalp. Fights free radicals such as pollution that weigh down your hair and make it weaker. Other Vitamin A rich foods include sweet potatoes, dark green leafy vegetables, squash, romaine lettuce, dried apricots, cantaloupe, sweet red bell peppers, tuna, and tropical fruit such as mangoes.

For healthy hair and beauty, food variety may be the best option. A balanced diet of lean proteins, fruits, and vegetables, whole grains, legumes, and fatty fish (salmon) and low fat dairy products are potential aides to hair.

Patient education

People experiencing hair loss should take appropriate advice from a physician, registered trichologist and registered dietician to determine the cause and any appropriate treatment. Whereas nutritional solutions may not currently cure hair loss, they may slowly assist its condition.

APPENDIX B

Hair Conditions and Possible Factors

Dry, Brittle hair – protein deficiency, possibly due to poor protein digestion; essential fatty acid deficiency; deficiencies in Vitamin A, sulfur, silicon, or zinc; imbalance involving thyroid hormones.

Oily Hair – essential fatty acid deficiency; deficiencies in zinc, Vitamin B6, riboflavin, or folic acid.

Coarse Hair – Vitamin A deficiency and possible hypothyroidism (vitamin A metabolism requires adequate levels of thyroid hormones); protein deficiency.

Split Ends or Untamed Hair – Iron deficiency; deficiencies in Vitamin B6, magnesium, or zinc.

Loss of Texture or Shine – essential fatty acid deficiency; deficiencies in Vitamin B6, magnesium, or zinc; imbalance involving growth hormone.

Premature Graying – usually related to stress; hormone imbalance (probably related to stress); deficiencies in B Vitamins, sulfur, copper, or folic acid; imbalance involving testosterone, growth hormone, or ACTH (a pituitary hormone).

Scalp Disorders (dandruff, Seborrhea, Psoriasis) – fungal infection; accelerated by a high carbohydrate diet; disruption of local and systemic immunity; aggravated by stress; essential fatty acid deficiency; deficiencies in B Vitamins, zinc, biotin, selenium, or copper (especially if sensitive to the sun).

Excessive Hair Loss – poor blood flow or poor circulation to the scalp; deficiencies in protein, essential fatty acids, B Vitamins, silicon, and zinc;

imbalance involving thyroid; growth hormone (especially if hair loss is all over), or ACTH.

Patchy Hair Loss – metal poisoning; deficiencies in folic acid and zinc; imbalance involving ACTH or cortisol.

Pubic or Armpit Hair Loss – imbalance involving DHEA.

Hair Loss on the Top of Head – imbalance involving cortisol, estrogens, progesterone, or testosterone.

Balding all Over the Head – imbalance involving thyroid hormones, DHEA, or estrogen.

*MOST OF THESE ISSUES ARE NUTRITIONAL DEFICIENCIES AND HORMONE IMBALANCE RELATED.

Bibliography

http://www.revitive.com
http://www.womensinternational.com
http://www.thehairlossclinic.com
http://www.webmd.com
http://www.hairscientists.org
http://health.howstuffworks.com

Simplifying Nutritional Wealth Series

A series of small, easy to read books addressing common health issues women tend to have through their years.
I have decided to mainly deal with WOMEN because we seem to throw hormones into the mix of everyday life. A lot of what we deal with and how we deal with obstacles comes from an emotional view. All we need to do is grab a hold of our hormones, keep them in balance and POOF…problem solved.

If we can understand the dynamics of controlling these hormones with nutrition, women will completely control the world they live in!! ENJOY!! Isra Girgrah Wynn

ISBN: 978-1-304-90891-9

http://www.iwynn.net

iwynn is a registered trademark ® of
iwynn productions, llc. and Isra Girgrah
Wynn.

Acknowledgements:
Thank you to everyone who supports
my vision, especially my loving
husband, Marty Wynn. And thanks to
my children who keep me on my toes
24/7.